A Victim's View

A "Victim's View" of Age Related Macular Degeneration;

READ HOW AVASTIN REVERSED AMD!

FIND ENCOURAGEMENT FROM AN AMD VICTIM IN THIS NINE YEAR DIARY OF LIFE WITH AMD; DIAGNOSIS TO TREATMENT.

by Emmitt J. Nelson, ME, PE

Mechanical Engineer, Registered Professional Engineer, Trained Mechanical Diagnostician and Amateur Personal Medical Symptom Observer

A Victim's View

A "Victim's View" of Age Related Macular Degeneration

December 2011

Published by:

Nelson Consulting, Inc.
10031 Briar Drive
Houston, Texas 77042
Copyright © 2011

by Emmitt J. Nelson, ME, PE

All rights reserved under International Copyright Conventions.

Printed in the United States of America

ISBN 978-0-9791685-6-7

A Victim's View

Foreword

This book is my effort to give victims of Age-Related Macular Degeneration (ARMD or simply AMD) some insight from the life of a co-victim of this mysterious and debilitating disease.

The word "Victim" is not used to sound as if I should be above such a health malady nor it is used to reflect a "poor pitiful little me attitude," but is used to reflect that in a real time sense AMD is happening to a lot of people and the cause is not known nor is a cure known. There is nothing that can be done to totally stop it from progressing as it occurs in a victim's life.

My good vision is gone with mere remnants remaining of what it was 6 years ago. As far as I know I did nothing personally to cause it. So to me that

A Victim's View

scenario describes the plight of being a "victim." Fortunately there are some things I can do to delay it and I will talk about those more later on in this narrative.

This story is not about a rapid cure nor is any medical advice offered though I will relate my experiences with treatment. But as I do this I am not qualified to offer medical advice but will from time to time offer my thoughts on issues a victim faces in coping with AMD.

This story is nothing other than me, a victim of AMD commenting on my vision loss journey and lessons learned on how to cope with low vision. I comment on how I have learned to live with the choices I have made as I travel through this new living condition for not only me,

A Victim's View

but all of my family as well, as all are adapting to my low vision as it worsens.

For instance family members are increasingly quick to point out walking hazards to me such as upcoming step-ups or step-downs. Falling is not of interest to me for I have done that, broken an arm and recovered. The fall was not caused by failing vision loss however but from not being alert to tripping hazards in plain view even to me.

Who Writes?

This book is written by a Mechanical Engineer (abbreviated as ME) and Registered Professional Engineer legally termed a PE. As an author I am not a Medical Doctor (MD) as are many others

A Victim's View

who have written books on AMD. These are easily found on an internet search in BarnesandNoble.com or Amazon.com.

This story will be published as a book and is printed, as you can see in very large type. The large type of course is on purpose because interestingly enough most if not all books on AMD seem to ignore the fact that the potential reader may be vision impaired.

That is not a criticism as most MD's who are indeed authorities on this vision mystery of mysteries are likely writing to other doctors or perhaps families of AMD victims; or perhaps to those in the very early stages of the malady.

Interestingly as one searches for AMD information on the internet many of the more alert web site owners/managers do offer larger type options for viewing

A Victim's View

their site. They obviously know many of we AMD victims are computer literate and may be looking for some magnification assistance; so for our reading ease larger type viewing is available on many AMD information web sites.

The books offered on the subject of AMD included few by victims so right away I thought; Aha, and asked.

"What is missing in this puzzle?"

Answer; "a book written by a Victim for other victims!"

Also missing was an account written by a victim of AMD using a large type that is readable by a greater number of co-victims and more easily by those who are not yet so vision impaired.

This work is being composed with computer soft-ware named "Microsoft

A Victim's View

Word" which allows for the use of very large type, even huge as one writes. When this manuscript gets to the publishing phase it will be easy to choose an even larger type, maybe even super-large size for the printer.

A good question that many who see this book in print will be, "Who does this engineer think he is, writing about anatomy and diseases of the human eye?"

My answer is first of all, I include as little as possible on the subject of anatomy; so my answer will be this; I write because; first I am human; second, I have eyes; third I have the disease AMD; fourth I am learning to live with it and; fifth I am a writer.

These five things, I feel easily qualify me to write and even justify my bravado as

A Victim's View

my vision loss journey and attendant experiences with AMD are recorded here; recorded in hope that these few words might bring a degree of comfort and assistance to others impaired with AMD.

Timing and Dates

The early chapters covering my history with AMD will be historical in nature looking back as what has transpired. However, beginning with Chapter 21 the narrative will be composed in a "here and now" mode, meaning that later in the book you will be reading of my experiences as I go; as they happen so to speak.

For instance later you will find me referring to anticipated cataract surgery

A Victim's View

and visits to a retina specialist. I recorded this visit as it occurred and then chapter by chapter you will find me writing in the present tense. In so doing I will give you indicators of the time lapse.

I began this work in early August 2011 and plan to publish it in January 2012. Thus the later chapters will be of experiences yet to be. In this way you can live my journey and experiences along with me as my path ahead unfolds, as the planned and unplanned events occur you can read about the outcomes as they happen.

As I go I will use the shorter form of the abbreviation AMD rather than ARMD. The later reminds me of the word "armed" so AMD it will be.

A Victim's View

Chapter 1

Age Related Macular Degeneration

The Disease

AMD is a disease of the retina. One can almost call it an anonymous disease, even though it has a name we do not know what causes it nor do we know how we get it. Physicians have found no cause to expect it is contagious so we apparently do not, by movement of germ or virus, contract it from others.

Medical sources do mention a few possible leading indicator diseases for AMD such as high blood pressure and

diabetes plus being overweight that "may be" (not totally sure) causative factors.

Like other diseases we identify AMD by the symptoms it causes and through physical examinations conducted by Retina Specialist Physicians who with years of education on maladies of the eyes using various "high tech" optical instruments peer into the eye, specifically at the retina for indicators of deterioration. Many amazingly complex machines are available to aid the Doctor in the assessment of the severity of our vision loss.

Since AMD is more common in older people (over 50 is used by some statisticians while others use age 60 to define us older people) the medical professions have labeled it "Age

A Victim's View

Related," but data reveals it actually can on occasion, again for unknown reasons, occur to people at much younger ages.[3]

The Macula

The Macula as a part of our retina is an area centered on and surrounding the head of the optic nerve. This area is the center of our acute vision and color discerning capabilities where our eyes detect fine detail that we become so accustomed to in our younger years. This specific interior area on the back side of the eye has been named the "Macula" by the medical profession.

Macula is a Latin word meaning "spot." Or in my terms the "spot" is the acute sight sensitive area centered on the

A Victim's View

head of the optic nerve as it enters the back side of the eye where it forms a circular area of special optic cells that give this portion of the retina our acute and color vision sight capabilities.

Thus the physical process at the cellular level that slowly erodes this acuity of vision is labeled "degeneration."

A Victim's View

Chapter 2

Can You Know if You Will Get It?

Reflecting

In truth, knowing what we do not know about AMD, the question is not, "Who will get it?" but is better phrased as "Who will find that they have it as they age."

In other words, due to family genes some will have a genetic[5] dispensation while "most" will not. I say most because only 200,000 people are diagnosed with AMD per year out of a population of 50,000,000 who are age 60 and older.

A Victim's View

The strongest indicator that you may end up with AMD is that an ancestor had it. Other than that single correlation, the available literature states that AMD is largely found in people over 60 who are overweight, who have high blood pressure and/or who are diabetic.

In truth no one accurately knows how many of the over 60 age population in the USA have the above indicators; nonetheless of the about 50,000,000* aged 60 and over American citizens a small percentage (0.4% - not 4% but 0.4%; a very small percentage) will be diagnosed with AMD in any given year, or some 200,000 per year.

So in any given decade about 2,000,000 AMD diagnoses will be made. While 2,000,000 is a significant number it pales in comparison for instance to the more

A Victim's View

than 35,000,000*** of the over 60 aged population that have High Blood Pressure (HBP). So one who is given to analyze the numbers can quickly see that if you end up, when you pass 60 years of age, with AMD, it is highly likely you will also be in one of the three groups, the HBP group, the overweight group or the diabetes group.

Interestingly, in my case two of my closest male friends, Bill and John each friends for over 50 years, both in my age group also have AMD. Two of us are a little weighty while the third is thin but all have high blood pressure but none have diabetes. John has an older brother who also has AMD in advanced stages.

Of the three John is a retired MD, Bill is a retired Children's Dentist and I am a "Still working some of the time"

A Victim's View

engineer. Though, I hasten to say that none of we three have actually retired, but simply have taken up different careers. John continues as a Medical School Instructor and talented after dinner speaker. Bill on retiring from the dentistry took up using his considerable talents as an artist to create beautiful abstract paintings.

We being close friends with the AMD commonality are into helping each other as much as we can. We have established sort of a brotherhood of AMD advice, assistance and counsel.

In my opinion, other than a few weakly correlated health indicators AMD, one's chances of having AMD is rooted in genetics more than anything else as oen ages.

What causes this genetic dispensation?

A Victim's View

No one as yet knows. There has been little research by drug companies but quite and lot sponsored by the National Institutes of Health, National Eye Institute.

Chapter 3

Is There a Cure for AMD?

The Answer

The simple and hard answer I have heard from the medical professions is; "No."

There are many highly qualified medical Ophthalmologists and Retina Specialists who are ready and willing to give you all the help that is available including some experimental work being done with cohorts from the general population of people who are first diagnosed with AMD.

A Victim's View

As you likely already know AMD exists in two forms; dry and wet with the latter being treatable. There are two principle drugs (there are a few others emerging in the market) in use to treat wet AMD; Avastin and Lucentis. The latter has been approved by the FDA while Avastin has not. Avastin was originally developed for colorectal cancer treatment. Though not FDA approved for treating AMD Avastin is being used "off label" as an alternate to Lucentis by most retina specialists for treating wet AMD.

Both drugs have been proven to stop or slow the progression of wet AMD. Most doctors have seen some of their patient's vision actually marginally improve with treatment of the wet type AMD.

A Victim's View

The injections are relatively painless and are given directly into the eye ball after specific drops are used to deaden the injection point. Lucentis is the most expensive and typically not covered by Medicare though that can change. However a few health plans do cover the expense of Lucentis but Medicare does not. My MD friend John is receiving the Lucentis injections into his right eye, though the AMD is not wet but the hope is that the drug will prevent it from turning wet or at least be there on hand should a wet condition begin to emerge.

In truth, since the population of AMD victims is small compared to other diseases of the aged there would not be sufficient potential monetary return for a drug company to search for and find a cure or a more effective deterrent.

A Victim's View

Even so there are a goodly number of Medical School Professors and Researchers who are seeking a breakthrough for least stopping the progression of the disease once it is diagnosed. Some interesting possibilities have surfaced in recent years but it is not my purpose to delve into these.

Suffice it to say; for now there is no cure available. There is the Avastin and Lucentis treatment route for the wet but neither uniformly stops or slows AMD in all patients. Thus a lot of research work has yet to be done and short of a miracle drug; we that have AMD can only hold out hope for a medical breakthrough. In the mean time we must learn to live with AMD.

A Victim's View

Chapter 4

Is My AMD Inherited?

Family History

A number of my ancestors lived to be over 60 years of age. If any of them had AMD no one ever mentioned it to me.

My older brother (87) apparently does not have AMD. Being a veteran of WW2 he routinely gets his eyes checked at the VA with no such indication.

Our father who died at age 59 did not have AMD as far as we know. Our mother did have cataracts at age 85 but never had surgery to correct the

A Victim's View

problems they were causing in her vision. She did have to give up driving but with close friends that could drive it did not hamper her activities.

Both my grandfathers and grandmothers and their siblings were largely farming families living in rural areas in Texas between 1875 and 1925, usually distant from the small town doctors available.

As such neither were they near any of the specialists of their day who might have diagnosed AMD if it had become a problem that caused a need to seek medical help. Some may have suffered from what was then known as Night Blindness but simply accepted it as an aging problem and left it at that.

If I had to guess I would say that some of my heritage group did have AMD but in the frontiers of Texas in the late 1800's

A Victim's View

and early 1900's it would be highly unusual for a problem to surface that would cause the seeking out of a specialist who would ultimately make such a diagnosis.

Summary: Did any of my ancestors have AMD; likely, but undiagnosed!

A Victim's View

Chapter 5

"Blind-Sided" by the Ophthalmologist

My Diagnosis

The background on my eyesight is that early on as a teenager I tested 20/10 and this drifted up to 20-20 until about at age 35 I began to have trouble reading. An eye exam produced a pair of reading glasses which I disliked and only wore when my eyes became tired.

Of course the chapter title pun is intended. But in truth as I have aged I have had no clue that I might have an encroaching vision problem later in my

A Victim's View

life other than my occasional bout with "floaters."

Floaters

If you are not familiar with the term "floater" allow me to explain. When the retina bleeds into the vitreous within the eye the blood breaks into small particles and floats around within the vitreous. These particles are noticeable moving bodies and are sufficiently troublesome to some people to cause concern. Currently I have floaters in both eyes.

My first experience with floaters was in the early 1980's. At the time I was doing a lot of flying in our Cessna Cardinal, a four place plane. At times I would venture into high altitudes to 10,000 feet. After these excursions sometimes I

A Victim's View

would notice floaters in my eyes. A visit to the eye doctor identified them with the advice to see an ophthalmologist if and when they became troublesome. It seems many people have floaters. I soon learned to ignore them except on one occasion in 1991 when they came on suddenly and densely causing me some alarm.

I rushed to an emergency visit with an ophthalmologist who examined my eyes and declared it a non-emergency. The problem abated in a few days and has never happened in that manner again. After that event I have on occasion experienced floaters which I have ignored as best as I could. When present they are particularly bothersome on a cloudy over-cast and gray day. In these conditions the floaters seem to be a lot more noticeable.

Vision Help

As mentioned above I first sought vision assistance at age 35 or so. It was determined that I had astigmatism and indeed needed corrective lenses. These I purchased but used little. Prior to age 35 it seemed by squeezing my eyes with what we call our frowning muscles I was able to sufficiently reshape my eyeballs to be able to self-correct the astigmatism to where I could see clearly. Some people call this "squinting." In fact this became such a habit that my friends often asked; "Why are you frowning so?"

Since I was typically a happy person I had no good answer.

A Victim's View

AMD Arrives

About 9 years ago after being asked if I wanted to have an eye exam co-incident with my wife Ginny's appointment; I said "Sure, why not. It has been a long time since I had one so we will do it together." It is about time I thought for I was now 73 years old.

The Retina Specialist Visit

The scenario went like this: We arrive on time at a prestigious Houston eye clinic. We check in and go to the waiting area reading our books to pass the time. Soon we are called together into the exam office. We both are met and our eyes are pre-medicated by the assistant and asked to wait a few minutes and the

A Victim's View

Retina Specialist would be in to examine our eyes.

The Exam

He soon arrives and in a very professionnal and engaging manner proceeded to examine Ginny's eyes as he took her through all the eye positions required to get a good look at the maximum amount of Retina. As he went through the process he made notes to his file and on finishing he asked Ginny to wait until after he examined my eyes to get a report on her exam results.

So in the chair I go and the procedure starts over again. Eyes up, eyes down, eyes right eyes left. Somewhere between eyes up and eyes down the doctor utters a comment; "Ahem,"

A Victim's View

meaning he is into new territory I assumed. He goes through the ups and downs and side to sides multiple times making notes and sketching little drawings.

The Good News and the Bad News

After what seemed like an anxious eternity he finishes, composes himself and addresses Ginny with, "Mrs. Nelson your eyes are in fine condition but Mr. Nelson you have an onset of Macular Degeneration."

At the speed of light my mind swept through a litany of questions of; what exactly is it, where did it come from, why do I have it, what happens next and am I going blind?

A Victim's View

Continuing, he described the disease and its potential to end in my loss of total central vision. He then in random order continued to answer all the questions; It is called AMD, it is likely inherited, we will need to frequently monitor for progression and in time the odds are you will lose your central vision.

Any more questions he asked? He kindly answered another long impromptu list and gave me this final information pointing out that my right eye was more effected than my left.

The Doctor's Counsel

Looking at me he continued; saying AMD is typically age related, we do not know what causes it, our experience is it will

A Victim's View

get worse, at what rate we do not know as the worsening varies by individual.

What you can do is visit your drug store and purchase a product manufactured by Bausch and Lomb called Areds. This over-the-counter remedy is vitamin based and has been shown in trials to delay the onset of AMD.

He further informed me that I also had the early stages of cataracts in both eyes and at some future date I might need to choose surgery to correct that problem.

As far as diet is concerned, the doctor continued we recommend you eat a lot of green leafy vegetables, the darker the green the better.

A Victim's View

As we departed we made our next appointment, me 6 months later and Ginny one year.

New Advances Since 2008

Now in 2011 the "nothing can be done" prognosis has changed so the advice from the medical community now is to see a doctor immediately when any evidence at all indicates your vision is worsening. If it is AMD then the Avastin/Lucentis options are available to slow AMD development in some patients.

A Victim's View

Chapter 6

My Take on What the Doctor Said

Remembering

What I remembered best were the words condensed by me: "We do not know what causes it. We do not know how to cure it but we do know this: It will get worse." Recall this was 2005 medical opinion.

As I absorbed this information I became both very concerned and somewhat pragmatic, knowing when the days ahead revealed the increasing loss of vision my life style would have to change. My interests would have to change and my liberties would be constrained. My liberties as in freedom, freedom to continue my life's work, freedom to engage in some of my favorite outdoor activities such as fishing and hunting which would be altered.

I determined that I would do the best I could to make whatever adjustment I needed to make to remain as active and involved in life's journey as I could. I never felt a sense of panic nor did the "Why me?" question cross my mind.

Areds to the Rescue

As a patient I began taking the Areds as suggested and have kept taking them to this day. At present I am taking two soft gels per day.

My personal opinion is Areds do assist; as the doctor said, they seem to slow the progression, at least in my case the onset of the disease has been what I consider quite slow over time, but just as the doctor advised it has gotten worse.

When you are losing your vision the term "slow" or "fast" is a relative term. By slow I mean that the relative progression has not been, for instance, over a six month time frame but rather has been over a six year time frame.

The Many Revisits

For the next two years I faithfully went for my every 6 months checkup and

A Victim's View

things looked good; not much vision loss progression.

The doctor advised to "keep the good habits up" and return for a checkup in six months.

A Victim's View

Chapter 7

An Engineer's Perspective

My "View" on AMD

As noted earlier I am a Mechanical Engineer and as such have, aided by my studies acquired over my 60 year career in engineering what I feel are significant mechanical diagnostic skills.

I define mechanical diagnostics as observing, classifying and correlating the collected information and using it to determine probable outcomes and causes. I recognize this diagnostic skill is not necessarily one exclusively learned as an engineering student for God created animals of all types with the power of self-preservation; especially the human species. This ability is illustrated early in life when as small children we learn that a fire or stove top heating element can be hot and touching it might cause pain.

The child gains through a painful experience the knowledge that, "the hot thing hurts so I will refrain from touching it." The child observed, collected information and deduced an action plan to avoid hurt.

Also studying engineering does not necessarily make an engineer more adept at determining probable cause for some non-professional people very quickly attain an impressive mechanical assessment capability. We say in these

A Victim's View

cases that the individual has a natural mechanical ability.

However studying engineering and physics does give knowledge of the laws of physics and mechanics to aid our God given ability to determine probable cause.

Similarly, studying the field of medicine gives doctors information on the functioning of the human anatomy providing them with the knowledge to discern probable cause of the health problems we have.

So I am not suggesting that an engineer is better at self-assessment than others; I am only saying that I feel it has helped me.

A Victim's View

Chapter 8

Personally Observing my Vision Loss

"Seeing" my Vision Loss

So it was a certainty that I would by my training and my nature begin to monitor my vision in any manner that I could. On one of my visits I informed the doctor prior to his exam exactly what shape the retina damage was taking over time. On completion of his exam I asked how my assessment compared to what he saw; His reply; "Very close."

I then asked the doctor; "Is the loss of vision caused by dry AMD an ever so

A Victim's View

slow desensitizing of the retina to where more and more light was required to see clearly." He confirmed that from a practical perspective this was true.

With the passing of time I have made a distinct correlation, the more light, the better my vision. To be sure, everyone's vision is less with less light but in AMD patients the vision acuity is orders of magnitude less. This "early on" self-determined fact aided my learning curve in doing vision loss self-assessments of a subject that I will cover in some detail later on.

The healthy human eye adjusts quite quickly when entering a darkened room from outdoor bright sunlight, such as one experiences on entering a movie. It normally takes about three minutes for the normal eye to adjust to less light.

A Victim's View

However the adjustment time required for one with AMD is significantly longer, in the extreme case up to an hour or more to fully adjust. Even then with the low level of light the vision will be significantly impaired for those with AMD.

My Vision Loss Assessment Process

Immediately after the AMD diagnosis I began to notice after retiring in the evenings that the rapidity with which my eyes adjusted to "lights out" was much slower than it used to be. This brings up the subject of night vision which was also getting worse with time. The time scale of my vision loss has not been a rapid one (as it could have been) but has taken some 10 years to this writing, from the age of 73 to the age of 82.

A Victim's View

My first self-exam clue or discovery was while looking at a gray carpet, closing both eyes for five minutes then opening my right eye (the one more advanced in vision loss at the time) I found when opening the eye a random circle of a shadow of darkness would appear on the rug. As I continued to stare at the rug the dark circle would quickly fade away.

At the time similar checks of my left eye resulted on no such dark circle. Well my question immediately was; why was the dark circle vanishing a few seconds after opening the eye?

The Eye/Brain Relationship

With a little internet reading I soon determined this is what the eye/brain

A Victim's View

function does automatically in such circumstances. The brain will, in a very short time span of a few seconds override the vision impairment and, in my words, paint all the area of vision loss background as the same gray color.

In fact, the eye/brain relationship is reported by the medical researchers to be so integrated that the retina in fact can be considered a part of the brain. Highly complex neurological processes are conducted by the eye as light rays fall on the cells of the retina.

I will not go further into this. Just know that we are possession of a most marvelous bio-electrical cellular system that allows us to view our surroundings.

If you are interested and are computer friendly there are many, many sources

A Victim's View

of information on AMD available on the internet.

A Victim's View

Chapter 9

From Dry to Wet in the Right

The Event

It was in 2002 that I was diagnosed with AMD. For two years I followed the advice of my doctor's and returned on schedule to be examined. In late July of 2007 the doctor visit took on a more extensive examination, more drops in the eyes and more tests. Some of the tests were done with brilliant light and were slightly painful.

Simultaneously with my eye problems I was also having some heart arrhythmia

A Victim's View

and as a consequence my blood pressure control medications were changed. The arrhythmia problem persisted so I determined the Areds may be conflicting with my BP meds (excess vitamin C being the issue) so I stopped the Areds hoping this might settle my heart down. In about 15 days I noted my right eye vision loss accelerated markedly as I decided it must be "going wet."

I was of course concerned but not alarmed as I remembered the doctor's words; "it will get worse." At that time in 2007 my doctor had not mentioned the availability or use of drug injections to slow or stop wet AMD.

So I became alert to the right eye and began to use my self-assessment process to quantify the effect of the

A Victim's View

somewhat more rapid increase in vision loss.

In a 15 day period there developed in my right eye a central dark shadowed area that fully covered central vision. My overall vision however, which is a product of both eyes, did not seem to be affected. In retrospect I now understand that what my right eye was giving up in vision acuity my left eye was picking up.

The right eye continued to deteriorate for a month as I closely self-monitored the progression. The central dark area grew in size over a 30 day period and then appeared to stabilize.

At first I did not at all suspect that my stopping the Areds could have been a factor in the vision loss in my right eye. Rather I immediately suspected that all the additional testing done by the doctor

A Victim's View

on my last visit was what caused the onset of the loss in vision.

I did restart the Areds after a month and concluded the heart issues were unrelated to the Areds, but continued to suspect the testing as the culprit.

The medical profession would likely say I was stupid to think this way and this may be true but as such it mattered not to me because you see I was still harboring and accepting the words of my doctor, "It will get worse."

My Doctors

With all I am saying about my doctors please do not think or conclude that I was in any way unhappy with my medical care. All who cared for me were professional and administered my care

A Victim's View

with the utmost in painstaking attention to detail.

A Victim's View

Chapter 10

The Biological Process Observed

Seeing Blindness

Please allow me to share this layman's day to day experience as I literally "watched" my right eye get worse.

How did I watch is the immediate question?

I would not attempt to explain what was happening biologically but will share with you what I could see happening. While this was macular activity was underway I often closed my eyes and simply observed what was going on in

A Victim's View

my right retina. As the biological process was progressing with my eyes closed I could actually see an amazing assortment of blue, red and green colors mixed with whites all continually waxing and waning in the retina. All this electrical activity was centered in the macula of my right eye. As vision debilitating as it was it became a daily habit to witness the splendored beautiful display of colors filled with dozens of micro-flashes of light per second on an ongoing basis.

When I explained it all to my doctors they remained quite casual and seemed to be fully informed on the subject.

I once likened what I was viewing as one might see a giant thunderstorm at night from 10 miles above it, without the color of course. The flashes of light were "pinpoint" in nature; not the "across the sky" flashes. When I described this to the doctor the reply was; "Yes, what you are seeing is the electrical activity in the retina."

Though I must say, unless a doctor has AMD developing in the manner mine developed in my right eye they really cannot have a clue as to how strikingly beautiful it was. I suppose one could say as evil as the sight loss is in the balance of things the beauty of the bio-electrical display was a distinct though certainly not a pleasant surprise given the gravity of what was occurring.

Dominate Eye Flipped

I had always been Right Eye dominate and did not notice until two months later

A Victim's View

that I had become Left Eye dominate. As mentioned earlier I am an outdoors type person and have done a lot of hunting; typically for big game where I used a scoped rifle. When a scope is to be used in my case, I am right handed so I place the rifle up to my right shoulder and view the target through the scope with the right eye. So the following October I made my annual trip to my local rifle range to fire a few practice rounds at targets 100 yards distant. In so doing on this particular day I set up on the shooting bench in my normal right handed position, took my seat and took a look at the target through my scope.

But surprise, surprise the target was not seen; instead all I could see was a blurred blob of real-estate between me and the target. Immediately I recognized

A Victim's View

the problem, accepted the situation and began a re-setup to fire the rifle left-handed. This took a bit of practice but it was not a hard transition at all, just being a little clumsy at first. I quickly adapted to being left eye dominate. It will be interesting to see what happens down the "vision loss road" I am traveling regarding eye dominance.

Chapter 11

The Radar Sweep

A Bright Light

During the days that of my right eye became wet with the accelerating vision loss I noted another phenomenon taking place in my right eye. This I called the "radar sweep."

It was during WW2 that Radar technology was unveiled. Radar development scientists used a Cathode Ray tube to register the reflection from powerful radio signals sent from a rotating transmitter/receiver antenna swept the

A Victim's View

sky in a 360 degree circle. Any airborne object the radio beam came in contact with will actually reflect the transmitted signal back to a return signal receiver. The output from the receiver was displayed on a Cathode Ray screen. The transmitter/receiver was a device that rotated at 12.5 RPM, or "rotations per minute." Each time the transmitter made a revolution it was called a sweep; as in sweeping the skies for a reflective object, which during WW2 was typically an aircraft. Equipped with this device the radar operator user could have an early warning of approaching aircraft.

This sweeping system, though much improved, is still in use today for military defense and is used as a tool of air traffic controllers around the world.

A Victim's View

Back to my right eye; what I was seeing as the accelerated vision loss was occurring and I still see many times each day in my right eye is the rather frequent flashes of light small in diameter sweeping counter clockwise. They last less than one second and are centered exactly on the retina where I would think the macula is situated.

When I asked my doctor about this they acknowledged that indeed this was a true event that can occur to an AMD victim.

In lay terms it seems the brain/retina senses that the right eye is transmitting garbage as far as normal retina bio-electrical transmission is concerned and the brain on occasion will overrule the transmission process and call for an over-riding vision sweep. This sweep is

A Victim's View

in effect the brain saying "Hey I am getting garbage here, where is the true picture?" Seeking the true picture it overrides the ongoing flawed signal system electrical input and implements a checking sweep seeking good data.

I know the above description will be laughable to the learned medical and radar professional, and that is ok with me.

This is not a medical book, but the words of a layman who has AMD and trying to describe to a fellow victim one of the many experiences AMD has unveiled in my life.

I wish to add before I leave this subject that there are "flashes of light" that occur in the eye that are of grave concern because when a retina is becoming detached the patient will see

A Victim's View

flashes of light. So do not ignore the random flashes of light that can occur and do report them to your doctor as I did.

A Victim's View

Chapter 12

Giving up Driving

Big Decision Time

Personal transportation has always been a major priority in America dating from the first settlers. The use of horse and mule animal power for traveling even short distances preceded the advent of the automobile. In 1900 most of America was existing in an agricultural society.

People were gaining a livelihood using animals; farming, moving cargo and people across this great land existing in

A Victim's View

an animal power based economy. Other than the waterways for travel in 1900 there were more horses and mules in America used for transportation. There were more animals than there were people by a large margin.

Every man and family had their own horses, mules and wagons. Even as late as 1932 when my father and mother moved to a new job for my parents even as a small child I remember we moved in a wagon drawn by a team of mules.

I am saying all this about personal transportation to say Americans have historically been accustomed to having personal transportation. It was every man a horse in the 19th century. This "every man a horse" has changed with the invention of the automobile to "every

A Victim's View

man, woman and teenager an automobile" in the 20th century.

The car population replaced the horse/mule/ oxen population to where today most families have more than one automobile just as earlier every family had more than one horse.

We folks in the older population here in 2011 of the 21st Century have become accustomed to being <u>singularly independent</u> which means we all have our own car. We can move at will. Just step out of our home, mount our auto and drive away. Away to where-ever, be it a 1000 mile journey or a 500 yard trip to our local Starbucks.

A Victim's View

Giving up Independence

So when a person of age has to contemplate giving up that kind of transportation independence it quickly becomes a life changing decision. All of a sudden we are no longer so independent but are now dependent. This change is softened in impact if you have a spouse who still has the faculties to drive. If not then you can be dramatically anchored to one spot.

It is then only by the good graces of children, grand-children or friends that you are able to move around in your neighborhood at all. The day you have to give up driving because of your AMD is a in a word, traumatic!

But give up this freedom many of we victims must; so prepare yourself and

A Victim's View

you will find it is not the end of the world after all.

AMD and Road Safety

It is easy to conclude AMD patients have a moral obligation to themselves, their family and to society to monitor their vision loss and make a "pre-next driver's license vision test" decision to curtail or even give up driving for their own sake and for the sake of the neighbor's safety.

I realize there are times when older drivers may be unaware of the progresssive nature of their own loss of vision acuity. This is what happened to my mother at age 84.

Mom was always a good driver having started at the age of 14 driving my grandfather around their farming com-

A Victim's View

munity in their Model T Ford car. As a matter of fact because she was so dependable granddad never learned to drive an automobile and he died at age 75 in 1950. In his last 10 years of life he reverted to horses and a wagon to travel the two miles of dirt road to the grocery in their local Texas farming community.

To continue Mom's story, in 1988 she and a friend went out in our small home town on a shopping trip. Mom was doing the driving, even though the automobile belonged to the friend. After stopping at a store to shop, on pulling out onto the highway they were broadsided by an oncoming car. The friend was uninjured but Mom's pelvis was broken. Interestingly neither Mom nor her friend saw the oncoming car, though both said were looking.

A Victim's View

She recovered in time and was again driving when shortly after when her driver's license came up for renewal it required a vision test. She went in to renew and promptly failed the vision test. She immediately went to her eye doctor who informed her she had a significant cataract in each eye and they needed removing and furthermore he could remove the first one tomorrow.

Here is the point; neither Mom, nor I or my older brother had any idea she had a vision problem.

With this news of cataracts she called me and I traveled the 30 miles to her home and we talked about her options. My brother and I were already discussing how we could get her to give up driving but had reached no decisions. As she related to me her options on surgery

A Victim's View

I asked her if she really wanted to go through with the eye surgery where upon, without hesitation replied she did not.

She said her friends would be happy to drive the cars they needed to get about town.

Problem solved.

Point is – She was not diagnosed with AMD but she did have a significant unknown vision problem.

In my case I figure do my-self and my community a favor. I am carefully monitoring my vision loss so I can make timely judgments for giving up driving. If it is cataracts then eye surgery is always an option. If it is AMD then I will choose giving up driving before I fail my eye test.

A Victim's View

Where am I in this Decision?

Persons with AMD and the vision loss will experience issues with family members during the time just prior to giving up driving.

All know I am impaired; the problem is they do not know just how impaired; only I know that information.

So I figure it is a good idea is to have family member passengers give me road vision tests. I even invite them to do so. For instance reading road signs and estimating the distance to the sign as it comes into reading clarity.

Otherwise what I will have is very frightened passengers shouting at me to "look out" for this or that when in fact I am seeing all and in perfect control. My strong conviction is to pleasantly endure

A Victim's View

this assistance and even welcome it reassuring them that I am ok with the help, even welcome it.

On the other hand I work to be very careful to know my own limitations. For instance, in my case I am aware that my vision loss is more extreme at night and near dusk. At these times I have difficulty seeing in the growing shadows along forested roads, especially in seeing the color red, especially stop sign red.

So what have I done about it? I drive very little. The driving I do which at this time is perfectly safe is limited to broad sunny daylight and around our very familiar neighborhoods where I am acquainted with stop sign locations. As I do this I concentrate on any shadows seeking to spot items that may not be so visible to me.

To illustrate my practice mentioned above, as I have begun to limit my driving one of the things I have done is to point out various objects that I can see alerting any family members riding with me what I could see so they were not totally uninformed and in effect riding on pins and needles.

At this writing I am very limited on what I can read in speed limit signs and signs with messages on them. The reading of street signs is almost a thing of the past with me. Consequently I am doing very little driving that is dependent on that skill. What driving I still do is extremely limited to my local highly familiar area and then only in bright daylight.

A Victim's View

My next driver's vision test will be June of 2012. Unless my planned cataract surgery provides me with significantly improved vision I will not even take the test but just apply for a picture identification card.

At present I am blessed with my wife Ginny age 76 who has no vision loss, in fact does not even wear glasses except to read, who is also a very good driver.

A Victim's View

Chapter 13

Scary Thoughts About Driving

Being Careful

One of the things Ginny and I have often discussed as we are edging ever older and wanting to remain independent as a couple is to be very safe as we drive. Just one bad accident and it could be we would lose our insurance. This of course would be the lesser of the evils as because if a car accident ever occurred it has the potential to cause hurt or even death to others not to mention one or both of us. As a consequence we often discuss this with each other to "keep us on our toes."

A Rain Storm Scares Us

On a June trip from Houston to Dallas to visit our grandson Pierce on his birthday we left Dallas near dark with plans to spend the night in a hotel south of Dallas about an hour's drive. All went well with Ginny driving until about 30 miles from our destination we could see a large thunderstorm with lots of lightening directly in our path. We discussed what to do and were hoping we could get to our hotel before we got into the rain.

Well, we almost made it; about three miles from our destination we encountered the rain; heavy rain. We did fine until we began our search for the exit off

A Victim's View

the Interstate. Ginny kept slowing down to see better in the downpour. Eighteen wheelers were zipping by us on our left as we poked along. Had it not been for my keen familiarity with the location of the exit we would have missed it.

The truth is we were scared and after this experience we promised ourselves to never do that again. It was a dark night, it was raining, we were in traffic and unsure; all summing to a dangerous combination.

Our decision was no more night driving on interstates in the rain. Later we modified that to no more night driving.

"What Ifs" Examined

Living in the Houston area for 22 years we are very familiar with the streets on

A Victim's View

our side of town so we can have a safe night outing in no rain conditions with Ginny driving in our part of the city.

But as for me it was in April I had some work to do about 60 miles from our home. It is Interstate all the way so I had no problem for me to drive the distance. For a few years now I have been leaving plenty of room between me and the car in front of me to adjust to aging reaction times.

The scene: It is a bright day and I am at 55 mile per hour in the right lane of the Interstate doing a good job keeping my distance. Then all of a sudden I note the Eighteen Wheeler in front of me is growing much larger at a very rapid pace. Belatedly apparent to me was that the truck was stopped. Since I was

A Victim's View

giving lots of following distance I had no trouble stopping but "what if?"

Later that Same Trip

The scene continues: As I close in on my arrival at my destination on the above trip I am on a two lane city street with no sidewalks. Instead there are drainage ditches on each side of the street with little to no shoulder room to move onto if needed. Had I been distracted by some little something I would not have seen the man in a motorized wheel chair in my lane traveling in the same direction. But notice him I did and eased around him on a "no traffic around" street.

You know how often drivers say on the subject of motorcycles; "I simply did not see it coming." How much smaller is a

A Victim's View

motorized wheel chair than a motor cycle? All I can say is the man in the wheel chair was engaging in risky behavior and for his safety counting on drivers being clear of eye and unimpaired in other ways.

As I reflected on this "what if", the thought of what could have happened took me nearer to a decision to give up driving.

Same Area a Week Later

I was to attend an early morning meeting in the same city a week later. By this time I had made the decision to avoid night driving when possible, when shadows are long and dusk lighting conditions prevail.

A Victim's View

On this occasion Ginny and I left home with me driving around 3pm to get ahead of the predictable rush hour traffic for the 60 mile journey. We also planned to spend the night in a local hotel so to avoid night driving home and the early rush hour traffic the next morning. On arrival we decided to eat dinner in a local sea food restaurant.

We stopped in the restaurant to have dinner before making our way to our motel. As it happened we found ourselves leaving the restaurant just at sundown. I chose to do the driving the short distance to the hotel. Stopping at a traffic light I chose to turn right on red (legal in Texas)and after checking to ensure the way was clear I proceeded into the turn only to be startled by the appearance of a small "red" sedan

A Victim's View

zooming by our vehicle. My immediate realization was, "hey, I did not see that car approaching," thus could have easily collided with it.

What was the issue? In my case as I mentioned above a color very difficult to see in poor light is red.

Conclusion: It was a bad decision for me to be driving in those evening lighting conditions. Ginny should have been in the driver's seat.

Chapter 14

Age 82 and Still Working

Blessed

The work I mentioned in the above paragraph causes me to realize that I am exceedingly blessed to have an extended career and I hope with God's help to continue to extend it. When I graduated from Engineering School in 1952 I took a job with Shell Oil Company as an Engineer in Training. My career with Shell was a gratifying one and when I retired in 1989 and looked back on those 37+ years I was content with what I saw. I had been trusted with much and found faithful and true. There could not

A Victim's View

have been a greater group of men and women to work with. It had been a fun filled time of challenge and success.

As good fortune would have it I was asked to continue my work as an independent consultant for Shell following retirement. This lasted four more years, during which time I learned a lot about construction safety.

Without getting into more detail, in 1990 I began my second career for the next 20+ years as a safety consultant teaching the art of safety leadership to corporate management with emphasis in the construction contractor world of commerce.

Nelson Consulting, Inc. was founded in the spring of 1992 and it has been an enjoyable extended career as I have assisted companies around the USA in

A Victim's View

establishing corporate safety cultures for the 21st Century.

The business model required that I do a lot of seminar speaking. The preparation work I did was done using computers so my ability to conduct my business became heavily dependent on the use of computer software.

During the period from 1996 to 2011, during my spare time I also continued my interest in writing and became an independent publisher causing me to be even more dependent on my computers.

I have authored nine books and many technical papers for trade magazines, most of that being on the subject of construction safety. As far as being a publisher is concerned I refer to the enterprise as my "vanity press." Only two of my nine books have sold a significant number of copies and these were the books on Safety. But they all are for sale and what funds I do get is considered corporate income.

Extended Career For How Long

The current big question in my life is; will I be able to continue working and if so for how long? If able then, what can I do to extend my working years with the tools I have become so dependent upon, my computers?

I have often pondered my future and sought advice from Bill and John and from other friends who have had family members with **AMD**. I consider any experienced based in put valuable and potentially usable as I travel my journey.

A Victim's View

Help From my Friends

My friend Bill, the retired Children's Dentist and co-victim of AMD has been surviving his radical loss of vision with his "never give up attitude." Bill sought out the Veteran's Administration (VA) and they proved more than willing to assist him with his vision problems. He discovered that the VA had a high tech computer based service for veterans with vision impairment. The VA supplies computer training and supplies computer software designed to enlarge the screen image and other computer based reading equipment for the veteran.

Bill took a number of VA sponsored "in residence" training courses in how to use software for vision impaired veterans. He came home from these

A Victim's View

excited and wanting to share his knowledge with his two AMD afflicted close friends.

Available Hardware for Low Visioned

Unknown to the sighted world there is an entire industry with an abundance of help for the near blind; in my case an AMD patient and this help is as close as your internet connection.

With the advent of the digital video cameras it became feasible to design machines to magnify reading material such as books, newspapers and news magazines. For the vision impaired this is done using a camera support device; an elevated structure allowing a camera to transmit an image of an item to read to a video screen. The device can be

A Victim's View

adjusted to increase magnification to the point desired for ease of reading.

I will mention two that I am aware of and there are likely more available.

The "Elmo" is a device designed for classroom work that is easily adaptable to a home setup. The camera is mounted on a small structure allowing the reading material to be placed underneath while it sends an image to a TV monitor or a projector that a teacher might use. The camera allows the video output to be enlarged as needed to permit ease in reading. http://www.elmousa.com/

The "Merlin" is a similar device manufactured primarily for the vision impaired and is purchased in a single unit, It has a built-in camera and mounted flat screen TV. http://dakotalink.tie.net/lowvision.html

A Victim's View

If you have innovative skills and know a little about cameras and video monitors one can easily create a homemade version that would be quite adequate.

Chapter 15

ZOOMTEXT™ to the rescue

Help From Bill

Since friend Bill is so receptive to tune in on any vision assistance, he again led the way for himself and his two friends into the world of computer software for the low vision impaired individual.

Not long ago he called me by phone and excitedly told me all about software he had been told about by the VA called ZOOMTEXT™. He had been provided a copy and was tutored in its use by the VA. Bill could not brag on it enough. The

A Victim's View

software has an apt name for that is exactly what it does; Zoom your computer monitor by multiples of 1.25, 1.50, 1.75 and 2.0 then by the number will Zoom you all the way to 36x.

This gets to be a small problem for smaller computer monitors for most of your image is off the screen to one side or the other. But not to worry all you do is move your mouse in the direction you wish to view and "viola," there you are.

If you wish you can do as I have done, buy a larger screen. "Wait a second," you might say, "that can get expensive." That is true to a degree but to all our benefit the one thing that keeps dropping in price these past few years are computers, screens and TVs. This is a boon to one such as I that is a "new computer" chaser by inclination.

A Victim's View

I have of professional necessity been driven by my AMD to vacate the realm of small computer screens and have moved to 26" to 37" screens. I fully plan to move to larger sizes if needed.

Another feature of Zoomtext is that the software includes a voice reader. Just push a button and you have a voice reading the test to you.

A closing word on ZOOMTEXT™ is that at this time it is not available for Mac computers. But the upside of that is that for less than $600 one can easily equip themselves with an IBM technology based computer ($300) with a large 37" TV as a monitor ($229).

A Victim's View

The ZOOMTEXT™ Keyboard

Yes, Zoomtext™ sells its own version of the normal computer keyboard. It is no larger than many of the usual keyboards but has a number of customized keys. These allow you to enlarge the screen image with the pushing of a button.

I will say that I am not yet gifted in its various uses. The real redeeming virtue of the Zoomtext™ keyboard is that the keys are each labeled with letters and symbols at least 3/8" tall thus very visible to me. This contrasted to the normal keyboard key letters which in poor light I can hardly see.

The Zoomtext™ keyboard is available in Black with White key letters or if you prefer in Yellow with Black key letters.

A Victim's View

I have the Black but one may purchase a keyboard using yellow keys with black letters and numbers.

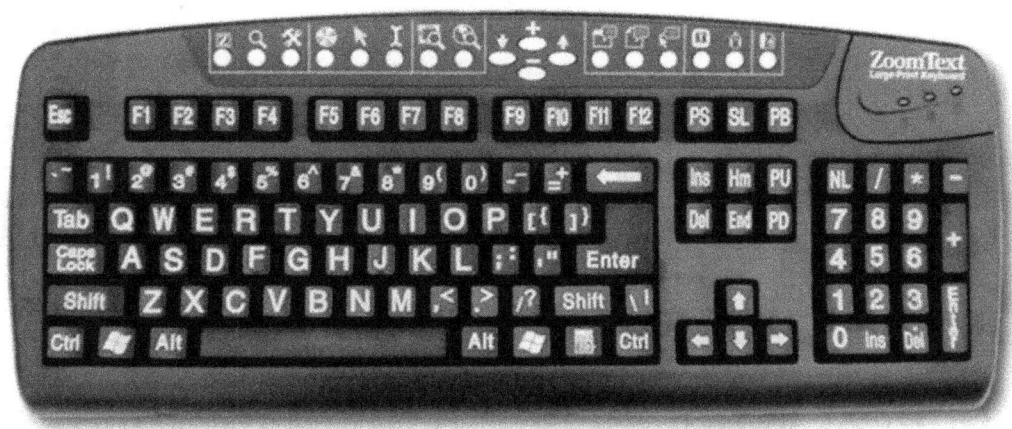

Chapter 16

Reading and Writing Still

Help from Zoomtext

Zoomtext is not so much needed while composing as I am now, however, when you are surfing the internet Zoomtext comes to the rescue. It takes the internet page material and magnifies it to your specifications, all the way up to "36 X" power which in a word is

GIGANTIC.

It is true that Microsoft Word software gives me the option to compose in this

A Victim's View

very large type even huge type if I needed it. You are reading 20 point type now.

If I so chose I could even write **in types this large.** But we will stay with 20 point. Imagine taking the word "large" and magnifying it 36 times and you can feel the power of Zoomtext at 36X.

Thus I do not need Zoomtext to read or write documents written in MS Word.

A Victim's View

NookBook™

One of favorite pastimes has always been reading for pleasure. In my early days of battling AMD I have been very concerned about how I can productively fill my time as my vision worsens. If I must of course I could give up reading and go to listening to purchased books on a Compact Disk (CD).

In the meantime I have discovered eBooks. A number of manufacturers are now selling electronic book readers. These are simple computer based book shaped devices into which you can install up to as many as 6000 books. Once installed – the technical word here is "downloaded" – you have access to them so you then can read the books in larger type about this size. Book seller Barnes and Noble has an eBook reader

A Victim's View

they call the NookBook™. I purchased one recently and really like it. It does have a serious shortcoming for low vision people for it does not enlarge anything but the book once you choose a book and begin to read. All other operations are in small print, so a nice magnifying glass is needed to find a book you have in the Nook.

The "Kindle™" iBook reader is sold by Amazon and Consumer Reports gives it very fine ratings.

There are at least 24 makes of eBook readers and with time like other electronics all will become less expensive and even more useful.

A Victim's View

Chapter 17

Back to the AMD Subject

Current Eye Condition

My "here and now" section begins here.

Both eyes have been dry for 4 years with the right having gone wet then back to dry in 2007 leaving behind substantial vision loss. The left eye has been holding up well in its normal dry condition "until recently."

With that said I believe I am now bothered in both eyes by cataracts so it is not an easy matter to separate the symptoms at this time except to say both eyes are getting worse. I do believe the recent left eye vision loss is due to the

A Victim's View

encroachment of the cataract. We will see.

Looking for Cataracts

The word "cataract" is word of European origin and means "obstruction," in this case, an obstruction in the lens of the eye. Self-assessing my left eye I can detect the presence of an odd shaped shadow around the eye center.

This shadow, if a cataract of course is situated in the lens and would appear in my vision as the blurry shadow I see so I am thinking this is what is going on. Past eye exams of both eyes confirm cataracts in both with the right being the worse which confirms my "self-assessment" process.

A Victim's View

Choosing an Eye Surgeon

Choosing physicians for me is a matter of seeking out friends whom have had the same problem and deciding which one to call on. For reasons of convenience I wanted one in easy driving distance. This search culminated when I found friends my age that had used a cataract specialist physician only a 20 minute drive away and had great success.

An appointment was made.

Checking in with the Cataract Surgeon

The appointment with a Cataract specialist soon turned out to be a disappointment for me. After a thorough exam in the doctor's opinion while I had cataracts in both eyes they were

A Victim's View

pronounced as only a minimal 20/30 impairment and then concluded my recent vision loss likely due to the advance of AMD. Having been informed of my AMD history the doctor recommended I see a retina specialist just in case my left eye AMD had gone wet but agreed to conduct a test for the wet condition using a dye to be injected into an artery.

On hearing that I would have to sign a form that the dye could cause a number of allergic reactions including death I declined, not because of the threat of death but because of other potential problems with the dye and other reactions. And in all my tests for wet AMD I had not had to undergo such a procedure to determine a wet condition. Net it to say I decided not to be tested in this way but in my mind decided I would go back to a retina specialist. This appointment was made soon after leaving the clinic.

Cataract Results

Concluding the cataract surgeon had diagnosed my vision issues in a responsible manner given the lack of historical knowledge of my condition with the doctor's area of expertise I now had more information. I received clear advice to see a retina specialist "next week" since it was already late Friday.

While I attempted to describe my personal view of my vision problems to the physician it was largely ignored as far as I could tell. This I take blame for

A Victim's View

this and have formed my approach to my next specialist.

You know the AMD sufferer's problem is the eye doctors we see have yet to experience the blight of AMD in their own vision. They obviously "see our AMD infested with any cataracts looking in; while we see them looking out."

In my case as mentioned my vision impairment has increased significantly in the past four months. Also as mentioned my AMD has been around a while in both eyes. The left has always been dry but the AMD vision loss has very slowly increased anyway which is what AMD dry does; slow and insidiously. Fortunately in this case though the AMD in my left eye has been off center (up and to the left of vision central) and thus has not impaired my central vision acuity

A Victim's View

that much. With this condition I have been able to function fairly normally; severely impaired in the right eye but have been depending on my left eye central vision to sustain me since the right eye went wet almost exactly four years ago. Shortly after it went back to dry and has remained so as far as I now know.

So my self-informed opinion is I have a cataract in my left eye as diagnosed by optical professionals that is now beginning to obscure my central vision even more. At the same time I can also tell the creeping AMD is moving into the central area as well. If it is a dry movement nothing can be done about that but there is hope in my mind; it may be wet!

A Victim's View

In my case having lived four years with left eye vision with cataract present I would like to have the offending cataract removed. With as little vision acuity as I have left a 20/30 cataract is not a welcome presence.

This is September. In May with my left eye a normal book or newspaper could be read; the right having lost central vision acuity in 2007. So for the past 4 years I have closely observed for any deterioration in my left eye. Since May it has been obvious to me that things were worsening. During this time I have been able to observe the forming of a shadow and have been hoping it was only a cataract. If it is, I wish it out. The retina specialist is my last hope.

A Victim's View

Diagramming my Vision Loss

The Sudoku square below is a good way to show the reader what my vision loss looks like from the inside out.

2	9	4
8	6	1
7	3	5

When I focus on the 6 with my right eye I do not see the block of 9 numbers at all. However, when I focus on the 6 with my left eye I can see 8 numbers with the 2 missing. The other 8 numbers are visible. This has been the case for the past four years. In the past 6 months all the visible numbers have gotten blurry. This means my left eye is getting worse. To be able to read, magnification is the answer. Bigger is better. My vision has been around a 20/80 in my left eye and

A Victim's View

20/200 in my right eye. If I could get the 20/30 cataract removed then I may be improved to 20/60.

The Big Question

Is the right eye "wet?" Also since it is true that such a cataract as I have will rob an AMD patient of 20 to 30 percent acuity it seems logical that to make the most of a sight losing situation the cataracts have to go.

The next stop is back to the Retina Specialist.

Chapter 18

To the Eye Clinic

Appointment Time

My wife and I arrived 10 minutes early for my 2pm appointment.

The Preparation

After a brief wait we were called into a treatment room and questioned by the medical assistant. Notes were taken, drawings were made of my vision loss opinions and routine vision tests were made. My right eye was 20/200 while my left eye was 20/80. Vision tests using both eyes also measured at 20/80.

A Victim's View

The assistant commented that my vision had not worsened since the last test about a year previous. The test may have so indicated but I knew better for there is a recent blurriness not present before. She then placed drops in both eyes and tested eye pressure which was normal.

Retina Tomography Photographs

Both eyes were then dilated and photographs were made of each retina. In the waiting area a few minutes later I was informed that the doctor had reviewed my various tests and wanted one more picture taken of the left retina.

This turned out to be a planned repeat of the test I refused at the Cataract doctor's office so again I gave my concerns to the technician who agreed and departed to inform the doctor of my preference. He returned soon and said the doctor agreed. We returned to the treatment room.

The Doctors

Soon there was a knock and a white coated doctor entered introducing himself as a Fellow of my doctor and proceeded to inquire of my condition and its history, conducted vision tests and examined my eyes.

He then gave us his opinion which was that I had wet **AMD** in both eyes and in summary recommended treatments in both eyes by injection of Avastin or Lucentis. He then meticulously answered questions regarding group testing of the drugs and gave us prices. I was astounded that both eyes were wet but took the news in stride but was far from comfortable and inclined to get a second opinion.

Friend John's Counsel

I was buffered in my shock by the recent experiences of my physician friend John who had had injection treatments in both eyes, first with Avastin and later with Lucentis. He had informed me that the process of a needle in my eye was a painless one and not to worry about any pain issues. He did explain that for a day or so I would have a "grainy" feeling in the injected eye as the needle entry point healed.

A Victim's View

John further had encouraged me to agree to the injections if and when my diagnosis came to that end point. While I trusted his judgment still I was both skeptical and concerned.

My questions were; will the drugs really do any good and what about a possible infection? Am I ready for that?

As mentioned earlier being a bit of a researcher I had searched the internet for information on the two drugs. Avastin was designed to curtail blood vessel growth in colorectal cancer and had some success in that application. An unnamed doctor on knowing that wet AMD is caused by the out-of-control growth of micro-blood vessels behind the retina came up with the idea of using Avastin as an injection to stop that growth.

A Victim's View

As time passed the news of the use spread and the drug was adopted by increasing numbers of Retina Specialists. This use was not approved by the FDA but the use persisted without it, called "off label" use. Reports of success soon prompted the inventors of Avastin to decide to develop a drug with the same curative characteristics of Avastin but designed specifically for the eyes and to seek FDA approval to market the drug. Over a period of years this was done and a drug was approved by the FDA named "Lucentis."

Thus the two drugs have become the drugs of choice by physicians who administer them by injection for wet AMD treatment. So I was not at all surprised to hear the recommendation from the Fellow. He thanked us and as he departed he said the specialist would be in shortly.

The Specialist Arrives

Soon the specialist appeared with an introduction for we had not met him prior. He did eye examinations and gave us his recommendation. He advised Avastin or Lucentis injections for my left eye and to do nothing for my right. Stating the testing of the two drugs had so far shown little difference in effectiveness he added that the cost Lucentis was about $2500 an injection while Avastin was $50.

Therefore he was recommending I agree to an injection of Avastin in my left eye that afternoon and to leave my right eye alone since it was already scarred and

A Victim's View

irreversibly damaged to the 20/200 level. This was right in line with my thinking after having talked to the Fellow.

Again many questions followed including his opinion on what was causing the roughly circular opaque obstruction appearing in my vision that I had determined was the cause of my recent increased blurring of vision. He could not say other than in his opinion it was not in the lens so it felt it had to be caused by blood under the retina. He showed me an abundance of pictures detailing where the blood was raising my retina off the back of the eye and again stated that he felt that this was the cause of the blurry circle I had mentioned to him.

So after a period of discussion and more questions by both me and Ginny it was

A Victim's View

decision time. I with some trepidation agreed with his assessment and his recommended treatment.

After even more questions about his experience with the drugs we found his answers credible for treatment of wet AMD. He said in his experience the wet form of the disease was effectively stopped by the Avastin injections in 80% of his patients, while 40% actually experienced an improvement in vision with as little as three injections. The remaining 20% see no benefit.

On the period of treatment he said that an initial 3 injections on one month intervals would be followed by more spaced out injections ending in about 7 per year.

A Victim's View

My Decision

My own assessment of the status of my eyes was that the left had turned wet and the right was still dry. So it was a surprise to learn the right was also wet. As mentioned above my left eye vision had been slowly but noticeably deteriorating for three to four months so in a way I was relieved to find out at last what was going on. On the other hand I was disappointed that my cataracts were once again deemed "not a problem," at least sufficiently enough a problem to warrant lens replacements.

The Injection

The preparations began at once for the injection. Three different eye drops were administered by an assistant over a 15

A Victim's View

minute time span. The most important one was to deaden the eye so the injection would be as pain free as possible. After an extended wait the doctor arrived once again and in rapid succession took the appropriate steps to inject the eye. With eye closed with a cotton swab he bathed the surrounding area in iodine to sterilize the area. I lost count of the steps he took leading up to the actual injection.

At last he brought out the needle and said "You will feel a slight prick as I insert the needle" and proceeded to do so. The prick came but not unbearable and the injection was made. As the fluid entered the eye I could feel an increase in pressure. He then said I would see a small black speck in my eye but not to worry about it for it would go away in a

A Victim's View

day or so. He also stated the cornea may develop a small area of redness but this would soon disappear and there would also be a residual stinging that would also diminish in a few hours at most and to keep the eye sanitary and avoid contaminating it. He did say I could use over the counter artificial tears if the eye became dry.

Ginny then asked if I could expect a vision improvement after this first injection. He felt I would in about a week or so. This I will report on later.

Later the next day Ginny made an appointment for me one month away.

Chapter 19

The Wait until Next Month

The Hour Following the Injection

We had arrived at 1:50 and departed around 5:45pm and headed to a nearby cafeteria for dinner. By the time we finished dining the earlier discomfort had diminished to the point that I was entirely comfortable.

In summary I would say the experience was not a bad one with only a small amount of pain in the form of stinging for about an hour. It soon stopped to where it was no longer noticeable. Visually

A Victim's View

speaking the eye was impaired with blurriness until the next morning. On awakening I found it no worse or any better than the morning previous. I was happy to find it no worse and resigned to wait over the next two weeks to see what developed if anything.

A Chronologue as I Wait

The word Chronologue does not appear in the dictionary, with or without the "u."

Not to worry I will define it to mean; "the product (record) of one recording a chronological sequence of events."

My purpose will be to self-examine my left eye to determine if the circle of obscured vision changes with time and record this experience from the perspective of the patient.

A Victim's View

I will let you know what transpires; my feelings, my assessments and my opinion; right now I am optimistic.

Dating the Chronologue

Since I am to have a series of injections I will label the day of the first injection as 1.0; then two days later will be 1.2. When the second injection occurs that day will be designated as 2.0; then the day after day 2.0 will be 2.1 etc.

Day 1.1:

On awakening this morning I examined the left eye by viewing the obscured areas that were clearly discernible as I looked at our bedroom ceiling. My personal eye vision exam showed no

A Victim's View

change from the day before except perhaps it was a little more blurry. This was to be expected according to the physician. As the day has passed I feel my vision has returned fully to what it was yesterday. At this point I see no improvement nor should I.

My Personal Eye Vision Exam Process

I do this exam in the following manner and it is very effective I feel.

There has to be some light in the room. On first opening my eyes in the morning I stare at the ceiling, first with one eye and then the other. What I see is only briefly viewable because the "eye-brain" connection will rapidly cause what I am describing to go away.

A Victim's View

Open your eye and immediately stare at the white ceiling. You are looking for areas of darkness or shadows. In less than 15 seconds if present the dark areas will fade away. The way you make them return is to close the eye again for about 30 seconds to a minute and repeat the process. I have done this for the past 6 years with success.

Today I feel all is well. No pain or discomfort with only a little redness and soreness in the eye.

No change in vision acuity.

Day 1.2:

The good news today is there is no apparent residual discomfort from the Avastin injection 40 hours ago. Vision acuity is unchanged.

A Victim's View

All is normal as the day prior to the injection.

Day 1.3:

All seems normal referring to the days just prior to the injection. There has been no change in the "circle of obscured vision" surrounding the macula. There is no noticeable change in vision acuity.

Day 1.4:

It should be too early to tell but I am "thinking" I can detect a slight decreasing of the AMD spot in my left eye; that is correct; the eye that got the injection only 4 days ago. I am a little skeptical but let's give it a chance for

A Victim's View

now. If I have to recant later then I will and you will read about it here. Even with this possible improvement all still looks a tad blurry but maybe a tad less than before!

8 5 7
2 1 4
3 6 9

Having said the above I can tell you that when I look at the 1 the 8 is still invisible. So what is it I am seeing? When I look at the 5 all numbers are visible. When I look at the 6 the 2 is missing. When I look at eh 9 the 1 is not seen.

At this point I simply do not know, maybe improve-ment, maybe nothing; we will "see!"

A Victim's View

The Power of Prayer

Allow me to "inject" here a little commentary on the Power of Prayer. Our daughter Julie I count as a world class prayer warrior. She is throughout each day praying for my vision. I pray for my vision and I know Ginny does as do many family members and friends.

When the wet AMD was ravaging my right eye I prayed earnestly for healing. Can I say that prayer went unanswered since my right eye vision measures 20/200? My answer is no. Who knows but without prayer it could be 20/500.

So as I go each day I place my faith in prayer and proceed. Do I have enough faith to make prayer work? I do not know but I have the Hope! I do know faith is a required part of divine healing. And I daily trust my wellbeing to God. The

A Victim's View

Bible says; "Man plans his path but God directs his steps." As for me I always want God directing my steps and I have faith that he does and will in the future as long as I leave it up to Him.

Day 1.5–1.7:

The possibility of the macular spot decreasing in my left eye is still in my mind for I am thinking I can see a decrease. I will report again on Day 14.

Day 1.14:

Possible good news! It seems certain that I have had an improvement in vision in my left eye. To measure it is hard but the apparent vision acuity improvement confirms my AMD effect observations

A Victim's View

made each morning on awakening. I would judge perhaps something like a 5% or maybe 10% improvement.

Obviously I should be elated and I am but reservedly so. I am grateful for any improvement to be sure. Every little bit of improvement is a blessing. But after all I am but a layman on things medical so it could be my imagination.

It has occurred to me that if in two weeks improvement is apparent then why am I on a once a month schedule. Why not two week intervals for injections? I will ask my doctor on my next visit.

The reason for monthly injections could have strong "medical" roots as a reason and it also could have a Medicare cost control reason. But if it were the latter the intervals for non-Medicare patients

A Victim's View

would be two weeks while us Medicare assisted folks would be four weeks.

But aside from that consideration there is the simple matter of the tending physician's patient load. If a physician has a fully loaded one month frequency for patient visits to change that frequency to two weeks for a large number of patients would place the doctor in a time constraint with not enough time to get all the needy patients treated.

Such improvement as I "may" be experiencing confirms my doctor's cautious encouragement. "You may see some improvement in two weeks."

So what to do? Cautious optimism and give credit to Avastin, my physician, prayer and give the Glory to God!

A Victim's View

I will file my next report with you at the 1.21 day mark. See you then. In the mean time I would like to again discuss and illustrate with drawings the results of my vision loss self-assessment.

Chapter 20

Illustrating my Vision Loss

The Process

It occurred to me that I can illustrate to you what I am briefly seeing each morning as I do my self-assessments. I have prepared two drawings for you, one of each eye.

Be reminded that each eye has a transparent yellow haze that surrounds the jagged circle I have used to depict what the retina is transmitting to the brain.

A Victim's View

I keep hoping the yellow haze is the effects of my cataract but I have not been assured that is the case. In talking to friends about their cataracts I do hear frequent reference to the yellow cast to their vision pre removal of the cataracts.

Left Eye Day 1.14

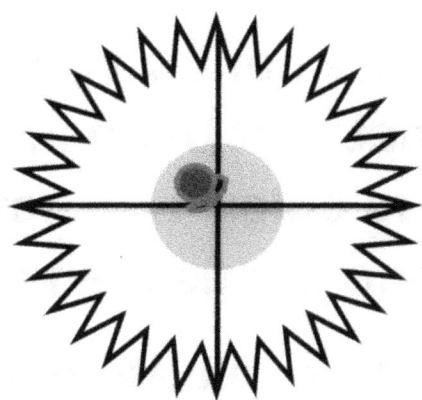

Current Left Eye AMD is up and to the left of center as displayed in the illustration. You will notice the two small wing like areas. These "wings" are of recent origin beginning to develop about

A Victim's View

a year ago and slowly becoming larger. Interestingly, however, none of the defined effected area in the left eye is a total eclipse of vision. By this I mean that these are the evident areas where increased light levels are needed to see clearly. Unlike the right eye where a larger central area is helped but very little if at all by increased light.

The larger circle in the center without a border is an area that first thing in the morning is a sky blue color. I do not know the significance of this if any.

Each morning as I self-evaluate my vision impairment I have noted since the injection the "tiny wing areas" are getting smaller. Please note that the impaired areas I am telling you about do not have clearly defined edges as appears in my illustrations, but are

A Victim's View

defined more it seems at the cellular level with small black dots of impairment that are the size of a "period" or smaller.

My thought is as the impairment continues to occur and more cells become involved the density of the impaired cells increase the size of the affected area and it becomes more and more noticeable to the patient.

All the above I offer as evidence supporting my belief that my left eye vision is improving.

Right Eye Day 1.14

Obscure

Total loss

Peripheral Vision

A Victim's View

My current right eye vision loss is central. The smaller circle of black is close to total loss while the margin out to the larger inner circle has some light sensitivity left and thus with more light the impairment decreases.

To give the reader perspective to my vision loss as I view the immediately above illustration some 18 inches from my computer screen with only my right eye all I can see are the word labels.

Viewing the same "right eye" display above with my "left eye" all that is obscured is a small portion of the jagged lines of the circle up and to the left of center. So it is my right eye that is keeping me going strong.

The net effect with both eyes open with these combined losses is very interesting and is a product I believe of the

A Victim's View

always present and marvelous "brain-eye" relationship.

With my left eye closed my right eye vision is blocked as commented on above but this "blocked effect" grows less as the light on the object being viewed increases with a remainder general blurriness in all peripheral areas. Remember this is viewing with my right eye.

With my right eye closed viewing with my better left eye the object being viewed is relatively clear with a fuzziness apparent on the upper left region as one would expect from the above "left eye" illustration.

8 5 7
2 1 4
3 6 9

A Victim's View

Regarding the Sudoku numbers above there has been no change. Viewing the 1 I see all numbers but the 8.

Explanation for Both Eye Vision

Now for the surprising kicker; while viewing with my left (better eye) with right eye closed an amazing thing happens when I do open my right eye (most impaired) the image improves markedly in clarity even though the object is totally invisible while using the right eye alone. The thin and transparent yellow haze remains.

The God Created Eye

God arranged this brain/eye relationship when He created one of the most

A Victim's View

amazing bio-electrical vision organs for our routine and "taken for granted" use. Now the human eye is not alone in the world of eyes. As we know most created species have eyes; usually two of them. You know of course the reason for two frontal facing eyes in humans is to give us depth perception allowing us to judge distances.

It is called the binocular effect.

Speaking of Binoculars

Did you know that patients with severe AMD can often see quite well using a telescope or a pair of binoculars? I am going to ask my doctor the reasons for this.

A Victim's View

Day 1.21:

Here we are on Day 21 and to use a pun "things are looking good" which is another way of saying I am convinced the single injection of Avastin has actually improved my vision noticeably. Things I could not do well prior are now accomplished with ease.

One of those is text messaging with my cell phone. As you likely know cell phone key pads are not known for being large in size. Well it had gotten to where I could not see the letters and numbers on my cell phone key pad well enough without a magnifying glass.

Also I note I can read smaller print than just prior to the injection. This I know for I have the Nookbook™ where you can enlarge the print to read a book, I can now comfortably use a smaller print than

A Victim's View

before. With study I can even make out the words in the Nookbook's smallest print. _{Which is about this size.} So all these indicators tell me I am some better off; maybe even a lot better off.

In addition and in support of these developments I can report that my self-exams are telling me that the portion of the retina in my left eye that is affected is slightly smaller in size.

I will give you my next report on Day 28.

Day 1.28:

Today as I awakened I was doing my normal vision evaluation staring at the ceiling and opening and closing my eyes seeking the AMD damage visible on the white ceiling of our bedroom when Ginny asked, "Are you checking your vision?"

A Victim's View

I replied, "Yes, I am." She responded with "How is it?"

This gets me to the next part. Since day 25 I have noticed the emerging of two new tiny areas of vision loss occurring. I say "occurring" because the way AMD affects the image my retina transmits to the brain is that it shows up in very small spots or an accumulation of very small spots. The spots show up almost one by one.

In the illustration below I am going to draw for you the image I saw this morning. Be reminded that these images I am speaking of are very temporary in nature as they will disappear in about 5 to 10 seconds with eye or eyes fully open. The two elongated spots to the right became visible in my morning evaluation, the first on day 25 and the

A Victim's View

second on day 26. As illustrated they are to the right of center and slightly elongated. Other spots surrounding the area of vision loss are even smaller and seem to remain static. They are about the size of this period "." and remain so. The two new ones are larger and are, as I said, elongated

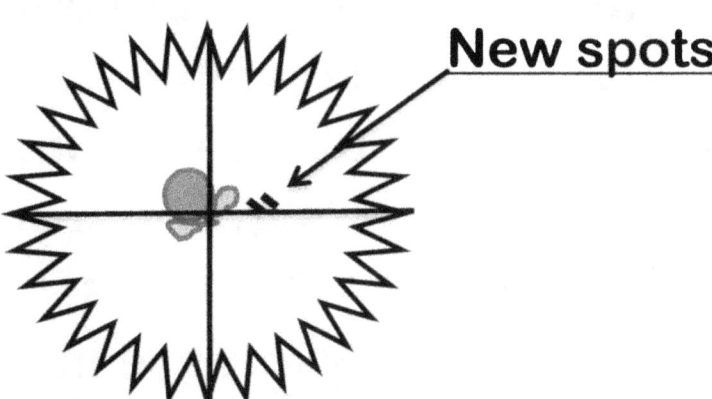

Left eye day 1.28

Recall at day 1.14, I reported the tiny "wing areas" were thinning out. This thinning has stabilized at a point approximating what was present six months earlier and as a consequence

A Victim's View

my vision has improved noticeably since the Avastin injection four weeks ago.

What these new developments mean for the long term remains to be "seen." I will let you know as we go. In 48 hours I am to get the next Avastin injection into my left eye.

My feeling at this juncture is that I am encouraged but at the same time anxious. Encouraged that indeed I might be correct on my left eye sight improving and anxious because of what I was "seeing" happening in my left eye in the last three days with the appearing of the new spots.

In the meantime I plan to relax and "see" what happens during the doctor visit on Day 1.30.

Chapter 21

Going for Avastin Injection #2

Appointment

With an 8:30am appointment Ginny has done her usual great job of driving through the city traffic for an hour and we arrive on schedule. Soon after being seated we were greeted by a super nice aid that ushered us into the treatment room and asked of any vision improvement whereupon I related my optimism that the left eye had improved and I hoped measurably. She made some notes and soon began the standard office eye test.

A Victim's View

As it turned out the acuity in my left eye had improved from the 20/80 to 20/60 and I was even able to make out 3 of the five letters on the 20/40 line. Cautious optimism prevailed.

Eye dilation began and eye pressure was found to be 13 in each eye. Normal is between 10 and 20. She said too high or too low gives rise to glaucoma concerns.

From there I had the eye photography/tomography examinations. This test produces pictures which reveal the back of the retina in stratified layers. The test uses light rays in a manner similar in principle to a sonogram. With these recorded images the doctor can determine how severe the wet AMD has become and evaluate the potential suitability for a second Avastin injection.

A Victim's View

This accomplished we were soon back in the treatment chair. As we waited I mentioned to Ginny that I would not be at all surprised to hear the doctor recommend that we give injections to both eyes today.

When the doctor arrived he was very pleased (even enthusiastic) with the positive changes in the left eye retina as could be seen in the pictures and as verified by the eye exam. He placed the before and after pictures of the retina side by side and commented on what a significant improvement had occurred since the first injection.

From there he turned the subject to the right eye and suggested that today we give both eyes an injection. This based on my apparent good results in the left eye implying that in my case for reasons unknown it may be possible to obtain some improvement in it as well. Needless to say I agreed.

At this point in the process the "hold harmless waiver" was produced by the aid for my signature. In print it pointed out that since they were about to perform an invasive procedure that could have a bad outcome such as an eye infection of even the loss of an eye it was necessary that I sign the document which in legalese stated that I had had these possibilities explained to me and that if bad things were to happen then no one could say that I had not been warned.

I signed the document just as I had prior to injection number one.

Preparations were immediately begun for the injections. This involved the administering of three different meds to both eyes on intervals of about 10 to 15 minutes. After this was complete the doctor returned and the injections were given. This time it was a painless process. Not even a little as was the case the last time.

The Injection Protocol Scenario

The doctor has assembled the pre-packaged and sterilized tools of his trade. First he administers another round of eye drops to anesthetise the eye even more. This accomplished he asks me to close both eyes then he swaths the eye lids, in this case both, with an iodine solution to kill germs resident on the eye lids. After this he places a small plastic like spring loaded implement that I will call a "spreader"

A Victim's View

that keeps the eye lid open in the eyeball to be injected.

Following this in rapid order he takes a large Q-tip with a medication on it and presses it firmly on the eyeball just where the injection is to be made; the syringe is then brought to the eye and the injection is made very carefully using both hands with one holding the syringe and the other pressing the plunger. The instant the plunger is pressed I could feel the pressure in the eye painlessly increase. Quickly then he administers a second medication to the injection point with a second industrial size Q-tip. The spreader is then removed.

In my case the procedure is repeated for the other eye. Once the second injection is completed he asked me again to close both eyes as he washes the eye lids to

A Victim's View

remove the iodine solution. This takes less than a minute and the eyes are dried with a tissue and it is finished.

Great progress he says and asks that we make a follow-up appointment in four weeks and bids us good-day.

The Injection - Immediate Aftermath

It is now near noon and we obtain our vehicle and proceed toward a favorite cafeteria that is on the way home.

Both eyes are extremely blurred since they have been fully dilated plus a foreign substance has been injected into both. Sunshades are a must of course. There is but little discomfort except with the severely impaired vision admittedly being a little distracting.

A Victim's View

After dining successfully through blurry eyes and with no food on my shirt I declare victory and we head home. A short nap on arriving and I am back at my computer telling you all about my day when Avastin injections #2 and #3 were given.

Chapter 22

The Days Following Injection #2

Day 2.1:

By the next morning the eye dilation was over and my vision was as is normal for recent days. The two little black spots were evident but low in the vision field so not bothersome at all. I had no pain. A little soreness in the eye was all I could say was a residual effect of the injections although Ginny did say both eyes had redness. Otherwise all is well!

A Victim's View

Day 2.2:

There is no change from yesterday but I do need to report that the small black spots that appeared on days 25 and 26 now have companion spots and a small area of impairment is beginning to form. Whether this is wet or dry I have no clue but it may be the latter. At present the area of spots is readily viewable on awakening each morning in my *"first thing in the morning self-vision evaluation."*

I did mention these new "spot" events to the doctor who had no comment. All I can say is I will watch and wait. I will report again on Day 2.7 unless something new happens.

A Victim's View

Day 2.3:

All is well in the left eye except a few additional spots were visible this morning appearing in the previously described area. Of note is while these new spots are quite noticeable in very low light they are quick to vanish at a very low but slightly increased level of light. I talked by phone with my friend John yesterday and he pointed out that he has noticed that it is almost like "no day is the same as yesterday" since he has been receiving injections in both eyes.

In thinking about it, a layman like me has to conclude that as the injections are being given the eye is likely benefitting. We have to remember that the drug induced complex biological changes that leads to vision improvement which are "visible to the attentive patient" would be unknown to even a medical researcher.

Even if a medical professional did extensive testing on a daily basis the researcher would be totally dependent on the results from the testing devices available to them. They would have all the testing information at hand yet remain unaware of the details of the vision change process the patient would be experiencing; unless of course those "patient visible changes" were the subject of the research.

Even then the researcher would be heavily dependent on the accuracy of the patient interview process and its success in obtaining information to use to correlate with the reports of the vision changes reported by the patient.

A Victim's View

As far as the right eye is concerned it has done fine with the exception that there is a residual soreness that still persists. I am unable to identify exactly where it is but hopefully it will diminish in a few more days.

Not all Patients Respond the Same.

Being an injection receiver and currently benefiting from Avastin injections in my left eye (the right eye response is yet to be determined; see below) I recall what the Retina Specialist said of the probabilities; about 80% will find a beneficial slowing or stopping of the AMD advance with about 40% having an improvement.

The math then says that 20% would not find improvement with even a few

A Victim's View

perhaps experiencing a negative response to an Avastin injection.

Remember the "sign here" form?

This latter possibility emerged very real from a friend this morning after I had mentioned my own "good news." She related how her mother was a victim of AMD and upon receiving an injection in her best eye it immediately became worse while wishing of course that she had never agreed to the injection.

While I was given the 80% rule by my physician he also gave me the negative possibility. Likely each retina specialist who has performed as many as a several hundred injections will have their own experiential data to recite.

Obviously a decision to undergo the injections is a very personal matter and

A Victim's View

only a victim's chosen physician after extensive testing will be in a position to make recommendations.

Day 2.4:

Left Eye:

The vision improvement is holding up well so far. For instance I have done a little experimenting with left eye vision and find I can easily read the following type size – _{read this.}

So to use a pun again, "things are looking good."

However, the number of black spots has continued to increase almost daily it seems. They are located up and to the right of vision central and seem to be very weak in their impact on left eye

A Victim's View

vision at this time. But I am concerned about their impact in the future. But so far I am fortunate that they are well away from the focal point of my retina. It is interesting to me that while the Avastin is actively reducing the wet condition sufficiently to actually have improved vision while at the same time added potential impairment is taking place. I suppose it could be the dry form of AMD doing its insidious advance simultaneously with the Avastin's reduction of the wet form of AMD.

Right Eye:

My right eye was damaged and even scared so long ago; 2007, that I am skeptical that any improvement will occur. On the other hand my vision seems better using both eyes. Even

A Victim's View

though the right is severely impaired it does seem to improve the clarity of the "left eye only" viewed object when the right is opened. Likely this is caused by the fact that though the right eye is impaired there are sufficient retina cells functioning normally to cause the improvement in clarity.

It may be that I will be unable to discern even with my vision self-analysis process whether or not it is improving. Being careful that I am not just imagining improvement is a constant effort.

Day 2.5:

Left Eye

Yesterday about 4:00pm I noticed something new with my left eye. There were about 6 to 8 tiny black spots

A Victim's View

scattered around in my vision field but not noticeable unless one stared at the sky. They are new on the scene!

At first I thought they were floaters but decided pretty quickly that they were not. The word "Tiny" leaves a lot of room for the imagination so I will attempt to depict in words how big they were. In looking at the sky imagine a black bird at 500 feet and you will have a close estimate of the size; not that big but a wonder nonetheless.

I can see three or four of them now as I stare at the white monitor screen; something to ponder.

Right Eye:

No change.

Day 2.6:

Left Eye

Today I am going to create another eye illustration of the black spots I spoke of earlier that began to occur on day 1.25. The shape in "top center" is the newly forming vision obscured area. As I have said I really do not know the significance of this development. See illustration below.

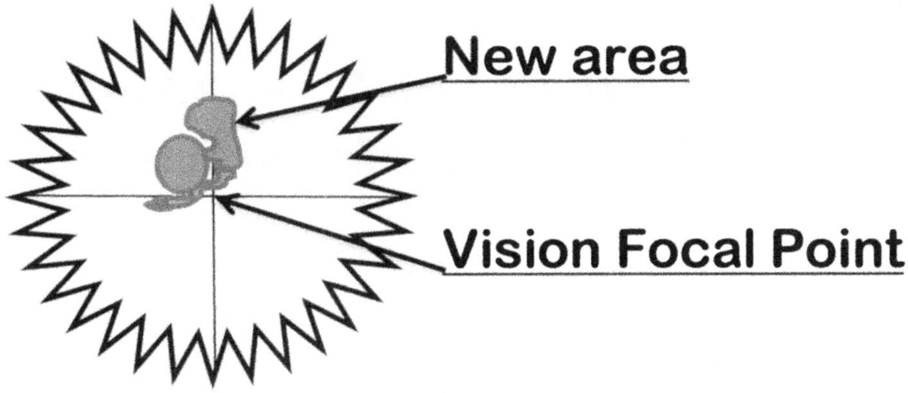
New area
Vision Focal Point

Left Eye

A Victim's View

Using an experienced based guessing process I am thinking it is the precursor to further sight loss. One thing about it that is of importance is that it is away from the vision focal point of the left eye.

Floaters

An update on the presence of floaters is that they can still be seen in both eyes; no better or no worse. As for the "blackbird at 500 feet" spots they seem to have disappeared.

Next report will be on 2.14 unless something changes of significance.

Day 2.14:

The "watch word" is "all is well."

A Victim's View

Left Eye:

The vision improvement seems to be holding up; no further noticeable improvement which is a "no change" report. The vision loss area remains static.

However, the very low light vision loss indicators are increasing and seem to be destined to encircle the entire area of vision central. This is the nature of AMD, wet at a rapid pace or dry at a somewhat much slower pace but ever so surely progressing. The end point in the left eye remains to develop.

Right Eye:

The injection two weeks ago to this point has resulted in no recognizable change.

A Victim's View

Day 2.21

Left Eye

Today is Thanksgiving Day and I have to say I am very thankful for the vision improvement I am experiencing. I hasten to add though I cannot tell if it will be lasting or not. Only time will tell that story. In the meantime I remain grateful for the progress.

My left eye, I believe is marginally continuing to improve. As I say this I am acutely aware that central vision in the left eye is a "touch and go" situation.

Yesterday I was on the rifle range with son and two grandsons. With the telescope I was able to see exceedingly clear the target and shot patterns but I was using a 20 power scope peering at a distance of 100 yards. The bullet holes in

A Victim's View

the target were just 0.25 inches diameter but very plain.

I am cautiously optimistic that the impairment in the left eye has decreased and is holding its own.

Right Eye:

If there is any improvement in the right eye it is not apparent in vision central. It was damaged too long ago and scar tissue is the problem. However there may be some decreasing of the blurriness of peripheral vision though I am still skeptical. Even identifying by testing the right eye is likely going to be difficult with a typical "read the letters on the wall" type test because the loss is so significant. I would love to get an improvement in the blurriness however.

A Victim's View

But we will see next week at the next doctor visit.

More on my Vision Exam Process

I have noticed as I have waited on my two Avastin injections to have its effect on my left eye that the results of the observations I am making day by day are very erratic. By that I mean each morning as I self evaluate the area of shadows in the retina are not exactly static day to day.

This was not the case prior to the Avastin injections when day after day I would observe the same shadow repeatedly. This is not to say I could not observe slow changes over time for I could. Over a few weeks I could tell the shadow was increasing in size.

A Victim's View

Nowadays I think I can see changes almost daily in the size and shape of the shadows. What I am not able to determine is whether or not the changes correlate with vision improvement or degradation. I have a feeling that it is likely both; that while the Avastin is working to decrease vision loss caused by the wet condition that the AMD is nonetheless continuing to slowly advance in the areas of dry AMD.

The last sentence introduces something I have not mentioned before. When an eye is diagnosed as wet AMD this diagnosis does not necessarily mean that the totality of the retina is wet but that some portion of it is. In some cases there are likely areas in the retina that are remaining dry. This would explain my personal phenomenon of vision

A Victim's View

improvement occurring simultaneously with continuing vision impairment.

While my vision in the left eye has definitely improved it by no means is perfect. I can read a rather small print book but with some difficulty as I must "rove" my eyes around a bit to pick up the total of the words to end up with sentences. This applies to small print only for I can currently easily read the larger type sizes.

While I can read a newspaper (slowly) I cannot read the type size used in a popular regional magazine named The Texas Monthly which uses uncommonly small type.

Ginny pointed out an article in the recent issue of The Texas Monthly to me to read yesterday but to read it I had to use my device similar to a Merlin reader. (See page 91.) It sits on one of my desks just to the right of my work position and consists of a roller mounted metal movable table top with a Video Camera and a high intensity light mounted some six inches above the table top. The video camera is connected to a 26" Flat Screen TV as a monitor. It was a gift from my friend Bill and it works fine for me.

The Yellow Haze

This is day 2.26 and it occurred to me to report to you the status of the current condition I referred to in Chapter 20 as a Yellow Haze or Cast. This Yellow area is present in the peripheral areas of both eyes surrounding vision central and had caused me to suspect it to be caused by cataracts.

A Victim's View

Here is some good news; the yellow has diminished noticeably and is no longer as apparent in either eye. In fact as far as the left eye is concerned I cannot readily detect it. For the right eye it is so damaged that it is hard to determine if the yellow has diminished due to the rather steady state of the peripheral blurriness which has persisted.

The question is; has the Avastin injection in each eye worked to reduce the impending retina damage that the yellow areas were indicating or is some other process at play.

Obviously I do not know for sure but I can say the intensity of the yellow haze in the left eye that was there before the Avastin injections is no longer as apparent. Only a small amount of the yellow cast remains in each eye.

A Victim's View

The deductive conclusion is Avastin may be helping that condition as well!

Chapter 23

Going for Avastin Injection Visit #3

Appointment

Ginny made the appointment for 8:45am.

An ontime arrival quickly finds me in the midst of all the testing to be done; Vision, eye pressure (L16 - R18) and tomography.

After going through the vision tests the technician advised that both eyes were improved over the last testing; the left eye from 20/60 to 20/50. The right eye was still at 20/200, but with additional clarity it seemed.

A Victim's View

Soon after being ushered into the treatment room after the tomography a "Resident" Doctor enters and asks questions and tells us good progress has been made. He stated that the doctor would likely recommend injections in the left eye for sure.

Soon after he departs the doctor enters and is very energized. He tells us he is excited about the tomograph of my right (bad) eye and the amazing significant improvement he sees since 28 days ago. He displayed the new and the old graphs to me and pointed out how much the fluid under the retina had reduced saying that if he had not conducted the tests himself he would not believe it, adding he had never seen anyone respond is such a positive fashion. I must say it was significant indeed.

A Victim's View

A sizable pocket of blood had simply vanished from under the retina. Of course Ginny and I are very happy about the report. He tells us the vision test in each eye showed improvement but more so in the right eye.

With that he again recommended injections in both eyes. We agreed and in a few minutes the "warning form" was sighed and the injections were completed.

He then asks me to return in seven weeks for the next testing and that was good news. I was hoping for a six week interval so seven was good news. He explained that such spacing of injections were common practice. That after a series of three (two on the right eye) injections most doctors set the next interval a six to seven weeks.

A Victim's View

Day 3.7:

The progress since 2.7 has not been dramatic but I do feel the Left Eye may be continuing to improve in a marginal way. In the Right Eye I do think the clarity of my peripheral vision may be improving some but as yet the injection has not made any detectable improvement in my central vision; nor am I expecting my right eye to be improved since residual scarring caused by the 2007 wet condition will be the problem.

However, all in all I am improved for which I am very thankful. Only time will tell how long the improvement will last.

I was talking to my friend Bill today and was telling him of my good fortune with the injections. From the start his AMD

A Victim's View

He told me something else about AMD vision loss I had not known. Being an artist he asked if I knew that the famous French painter Monet suffered from cataracts and possibly suffered from AMD as well. Bill said as Monet aged from age 58 his paintings became less "realistic" and more what is termed today "impressionistic." Bill said that it was due to Monet's and other artist's later in life paintings while vision impaired that "impressionism" came into being.

Chapter 24

"Looking Better"

Moving on

At this time I have reported on the first three Avastin injections and the days following.

The questions I face are "Do I need to report further? Will added information of my experiences assist anyone? Should I stop here and proceed with publishing?"

There will always be the creeping nature of the dry AMD that can "ever so slowly" take away vision acuity. Based on past experience with the passing of time it

A Victim's View

becomes very hard to decide if one's vision is getting better or getting worse.

A victim can only hope that the central vision loss that is the outcome of AMD comes on very very slowly allowing one to adjust to the loss and remain active. Maintaining activity of course depends on one's family and their availability to assist as the vision worsens. To assist with mobility mostly so one can live a reasonably active life and enjoy the living.

For me Ginny is always attentive but as far as my personal time is concerned it is the large computer screens and ZOOMTEXT™ that keep me writing. I now have a 32" TV as a monitor and fully expect to move up in size as my vision demands larger screens.

A Victim's View

Nearing Home

Of course at age 82 plus 5 months I am "Nearing Home" as the new Billy Graham book is titled. Only time will tell how it all comes out. My experience with AMD will continue until I "go home" so how does a Chronloguer decide when to stop logging and publish the work?

The answer in this case is; when enough information has been shared to be of some benefit to those who may want assistance in preparing their future path by reading an account of the high and low experiences one victim has had while traveling the AMD Highway.

Since the treatment of AMD will yield different results in each patient anyway, I feel it is time to stop writing and transfer the task from the writer to the reader.

A Victim's View

Below I offer you a closing Chapter of my final thoughts. As I am composing the information in the next chapter covering my experiences I specifically do not want to present these thoughts as recommendations; but offer them to represent my thoughts and feelings at this juncture in my journey into continued loss of vision acuity.

I do hope this work has been of some benefit to you. Thank you reading my AMD story and "Best Wishes" to you and yours.

Chapter 25

Lessons Learned

Medical Advances

The diagnosis and treatment of AMD has improved markedly in the past few years. When I was diagnosed with AMD in 2002 the outlook was grim. But thanks to the ever researching and innovative medical professions that specialize in eyes significant progress in treatment has been made for the AMD patient.

My initial diagnosis experience was rooted in the best information available in 2002 but by 2009 the 2002 information

A Victim's View

was significantly outdated and the good word was out on Avastin; and Lucentis and other lessor known drugs were introduced most of which have proven viable in treating wet AMD.

So far none the drugs have proven out to be a cure but can be a deterrent to wet AMD which robs one of vision at a rapid pace.

With the injections wet AMD "may" convert to the dry condition. That is the good news; but the remaining fact is the dry type of AMD remains a creeping nemesis to the vision of AMD patients.

According to current internet sources, studies and research on various treatments for AMD are underway by a number of professors at several medical schools. Some of these that I reviewed seem to be very promising.

A Victim's View

My final thought for an AMD patient is to "stay tuned" to what is going on in AMD research by scheduling regular visits to your Retina Specialist. Their job is to stay current. Many attend frequent conferences and read the professional journals on what is new in eye medicine and who knows but what the next innovation coming out of the research may save your sight.

If you are friendly with an internet capable computer and have the sight assisting tools I have mentioned above that are available to the vision impaired keep searching for the latest break through.

To my co-victim's I would like say that- "I wish you well."

End

www.ingramcontent.com/pod-product-compliance
Lightning Source LLC
Chambersburg PA
CBHW080544170426

43195CB00016B/2670